THE *Skinny*
5:2 DIET MEALS
FOR ONE
RECIPE BOOK

CookNation

The Skinny 5:2 Diet Meals For One

Single Serving Fast Day Recipes & Snacks Under 100, 200 & 300 Calories

A Bell & Mackenzie Publication

First published in 2013 by Bell & Mackenzie Publishing
Copyright © Bell & Mackenzie Publishing 2013

ISBN 978-0-9576447-4-8

Disclaimer
The information and advice in this book is intended as a guide only. Any individual should independently seek the advice of a health professional before embarking on a diet. Some recipes may contain nuts or traces of nuts. Those suffering from any allergies associated with nuts should avoid any recipes containing nuts or nut based oils.

Contents

Contents

Contents

Contents

Keep It Simple With Single Servings

So you've made the commitment to start the 5:2 Diet, or maybe you're into your second or third month and looking for some fresh recipe ideas for your fasting days. 'The Skinny 5:2 Diet Meals For One' is packed full of SINGLE SERVING delicious recipes under 100, 200 and 300 calories for your fasting days, as well as lots of SINGLE SERVING tasty snack ideas to keep you feeling full and motivated.

There are a multitude of 5:2 recipe books but most cater for multiple servings. This can be extra work adjusting ingredients to single servings – something you shouldn't need to worry about when your efforts are best placed concentrating on your diet. Just plan your fasting days around these SINGLE SERVING recipes and you will be on your way to losing those extra pounds and feeling great.

Each recipe has calorie information so you can keep track of your 500 (women)/600 (men) calorie fasting day limit.

The 5:2 Diet Explained

Imagine a diet where you can eat whatever you want for 5 days a week and only diet for 2. That's what the 5:2 Diet is, and it's revolutionised the way people think about dieting.

By allowing you the freedom to eat normally for MOST of the week and fast by restricting your calorie intake for just TWO non-consecutive days a week (500 calories per day for women/600 for men), you keep yourself motivated and remove that dreaded feeling of constantly denying yourself the food you really want to eat.

It still takes willpower, but it's nowhere near as much of a grind when you know that you have tomorrow to look forward to. It's all about freedom. The ability to be flexible with the days you choose to fast makes the likelihood of you sticking to the diet for a prolonged period, or even indefinitely as a lifestyle choice, much higher than a regime that requires calorie restriction every single day.

Popularised by Dr. Michael J. Mosley, the 5:2 diet plan has been adopted as a way of life, which will change your relationship with dieting and weight loss. What's more, this way of eating is believed to have major health benefits, which could alter your health forever!

How It Works

The concept of fasting is an ancient one and modern science is uncovering evidence that fasting can be an extremely healthy way to shed extra weight. Research has shown that it can reduce levels of IGF-1 (insulin-like growth factor 1, which leads to accelerated ageing), activate DNA repair genes, and reduce blood pressure, cholesterol and glucose levels as well as suggestions of a lower risk of heart disease and cancers.

In short, the 5:2 Diet works by restricting your body to fewer calories than it uses. Most importantly is that it does this in a way that remains healthy and is balanced by eating normally for the other 5 days of the week.

This book has been developed specifically to help you concentrate on the practice of 5:2 through our suggested single serving recipes. However if you want to find out more about the specific details of the science of the subject we would recommend Dr. Michael J. Mosley's work and, as with all diets, you should consider seeking advice from a health professional before starting.

If you are pregnant, breastfeeding, diabetic, suffer from any eating disorder or are under the age of 18 we do not recommend this diet for you. If you suffer from any health issues you should first seek the advice of a health professional before embarking on any form of diet.

What Will This Book Do For Me?

This book will give you a wide choice of delicious, SINGLE SERVING low calorie, easy to prepare meals and snacks that will not only form the basis of your 5:2 Diet plan but will also open your eyes to a new lifestyle choice.

The 5:2 Diet if followed correctly, will help you lose weight and in the long term, improve your overall health and immune system.

This book has been designed to help you through your 5:2 Diet journey by providing a wide selection of easy to prepare recipes and snack ideas FOR ONE to keep you motivated and your engine stoked during your fasting days. What makes the 5:2 Diet so good is that it's only a part time diet. Because you can eat what you want for the other 5 days a week, you'll be much more likely to stick with it over time and enjoy the long term health and weight benefits.

When Can I Expect To See Results?

By the end of your first week in most cases! Obviously everybody is different, but where someone is carrying extra weight they will normally see a reduction in the first week of embarking on the 5:2 Diet. Typically many will see a greater weight loss at the beginning, followed by a slowing down then eventually settling around a stable healthy weight.

Taking It Week By Week

The 5:2 Diet can work for you whatever your lifestyle. Each week you should think carefully about which days are likely to be best suited to your fasting days and then stick with it. You can change your fast days each week or keep in a regular routine, whichever suits you best. Ideally your fasting days should be non-consecutive. This gives you the opportunity to stay motivated by eating normally the following day, although it can be acceptable to fast for 2 days consecutively if you are feeling particularly inspired.

Of course, reducing your calorie intake for two days will take some getting used to and inevitably there will be hunger pangs to start with, but you'll be amazed at how quickly your body adapts to your new style of eating and, far from gorging the day after your fasting day, you'll find you simply enjoy the luxury of eating normally.

Whether you live on your own or part of a family, the single serving recipes will make it easy for you to stick to your fasting days.

How Will I Manage My Calorie Intake?

There are a number of different approaches to managing your 500 calorie intake (600 for men) on your fast days depending on your personal preferences and lifestyle.

OPTION 1: Skip breakfast, eat lunch & dinner.

OPTION 2: Skip lunch, eat breakfast and dinner.

OPTION 3: Eat little and often throughout the day.

There is much research and debate about the health benefits and risks of skipping meals, however the beauty of the 5:2 Diet is that the fasting occurs only for 2 days of the week with the remaining 5 reserved for 'normal' eating and recommended daily calorie intakes (1900-2000 for women, 2400-2500 for men). The point being that there is not a prolonged period of starving the body of calories, and eating balanced meals like those included in this book ensures that nutrition is still provided on the fasting days.

Portion Sizes

The size of the portion that you put on your plate will significantly affect your weight loss efforts. Filling your plate with over-sized portions will obviously increase your calorie intake and hamper your dieting efforts.

It's important that with all meals, both on your fasting and normal eating days, you use a correct sized portion, which generally is the size of your clenched fist.

This applies to any side dishes of vegetables and carbs too. You will be surprised at how quickly you will adopt this as the 'norm' as the weeks go by and you will begin to stop over-eating.

Measurements

All recipes are for one serving but can easily be increased if you are cooking for others too. As with portion sizes, stick with the recommended measurements of ingredients. Altering these will affect your calorie intake and therefore your ultimate weight loss.

Choosing Your Fast Days

Give yourself the best possible chance of success by choosing your fast days in advance and sticking to them. As we have already said, we recommend choosing two non-consecutive fasting days so that you only have one 24-hour period at a time where you have to concentrate on limiting your calories.

It makes sense to choose your fast days sensibly based on your own particular lifestyle. For example, for many, a Friday night may involve takeaway food after a hard week at work. If this is your ritual, then avoid this as your fasting day. Similarly if you meet up with friends during the week or have a business event that is likely to involve lunch or dinner then choose an alternative day. You can alter the days each week but just remember to check your calendars and prepare in advance.

Eat, Chew, Wait

In today's fast moving society many of use have adopted an unhealthy habit of eating. We eat as quickly as possibly without properly giving our bodies the chance to digest and feel full. Not only is this bad for your digestive system, but our bodies begin to relate food to just fuel instead of actually enjoying what we are eating.

Some simple tips for eating which may help you on your fasting days:

Eat. Take is slow. There is no rush.

Chew. It sounds obvious but you should properly chew your food and swallow only when it's broken down and you have enjoyed what you have tasted.

Wait. Before reaching for second helpings wait 5-10 minutes and let your body tell you whether you are still hungry. More often than not, the answer will be no and you will be satisfied with the meal you have had. A glass of water before each meal will help you with any cravings for more.

Nutrition

All of the recipes in this collection are balanced low calorie meals and snacks for one, which should keep you feeling full on your fasting days.

In any diet, it is important to balance your food between proteins, good carbs, dairy, fruit and vegetables.

Protein. Keeps you feeling full and is also essential for building body tissue. Good protein sources come from meat, fish and eggs.

Carbohydrates. Not all carbs are good and generally they are high in calories, which makes them difficult to include in a calorie limiting diet. Carbs are a good source of energy for your body as they are converted more easily into glucose (sugar) providing energy. Try to eat 'good carbs' which are high in fibre and nutrients e.g. whole fruits and veg, nuts, seeds, whole grain cereals, beans and legumes.

Dairy. Dairy products provide you with vitamins and minerals. Cheeses can be very high in calories but other products such as low calorie Greek yoghurt, crème fraiche and skimmed milk are all good.

Fruit & Vegetables. Eat your five a day. There is never a better time to fill your 5 a day quota. Not only are fruit and veg very healthy, they also fill up your plate and are ideal snacks when you are feeling hungry.

Some 5:2 Tips

Avoid too much exercise on your fasting days. Eating less is likely to make you feel a little weaker, certainly to start with, so don't put the pressure on yourself to exercise.

Avoid alcohol on your fasting days. Not only is alcohol packed with calories, it could also have a greater effect on you than usual as you haven't eaten as much.

Don't give up! Even if you find your fasting days tough to start with, stick with it. Remember you can eat what you like tomorrow without having to feel guilty.

Drink plenty of water throughout the day. Water is the best friend you have on your fasting days. It's good for you, has zero calories, and will fill you up and help stop you feeling hungry.

When you are eating each meal, put your fork down between bites – it will make you eat more slowly and you'll feel fuller on less food.

Drink a glass of water before and also with your meal. Again this will help you feel fuller.

Brush your teeth immediately after your meal to discourage yourself from eating more.

Have clear motivations. Think about what you are trying to achieve and stick with it. Remember you can eat what you want tomorrow.

If unwanted food cravings do strike, acknowledge them, then distract yourself. Go out for a walk, phone a friend, play with the kids, or paint your nails.

Whenever hunger hits, try waiting 15 minutes and ride out the cravings. You'll find they pass and you can move on with your day.

Remember - feeling hungry is not a bad thing. We are all so used to acting on the smallest hunger pangs that we forget what it's like to feel genuinely hungry. Feeling hungry for a couple of days a week is not going to harm you. Learn to 'own' your hunger and take control of how you deal with it.

If you feel you can't do it by yourself then get some support. Encourage a friend or partner to join you on the 5:2 Diet. Having someone to talk things through with can be a real help.

Get moving. Being active isn't a necessity for the 5:2 Diet to have results but as with all diets increased activity will complement your weight loss efforts. Think about what you are doing each day: choose the stairs instead of the lift, walk to the shops instead of driving. Making small changes will not only help you burn calories but will make you feel healthier and more in control of your weight loss.

Don't beat yourself up! If you have a bad day forget about it, don't feel guilty. Recognise where you went wrong and move on. Tomorrow is a new day and you can start all over again. Fast for just two days a week and you'll see results. Guaranteed!

Calorie Conscious Side Suggestions

If you want to make any of the recipes or snacks in this book more substantial you may want to add an accompaniment to them. Here's a list of some key side vegetables, salad, noodles etc which you may find useful when working out your calories.

All calories are per 100g/3 ½ oz Rice and noodle measurements are cooked weights

Asparagus: 20 cals

Beansprouts: 30 cals

Brussel Sprouts: 42 cals

Butternut Squash: 45 cals

Cabbage: 30 cals

Carrots: 41 cals

Cauliflower: 25 cals

Celery: 14 cals

Courgette/zucchini: 16 cals

Cucumber: 15 cals

Egg noodles: 62 cals

Green beans: 81 cals

Leeks: 61 cals

Long grain rice: 140 cals

Mixed salad leaves: 17 cals

Mixed salad leaves: 30 cals

Mushrooms: 22 cals

Pak choi; 13 cals

Parsnips: 67 cals

Peas: 64 cals

Pepper (bell): 20 cals

Potatoes: 75 cals

Rocket: 17 cals

Shirataki 'Miracle' noodles: 30 cals

Spinach: 23 cals

Sweet Potato: 86 cals

Sweet corn: 86 cals

Tomatoes: 18 cals

Skinny
5:2 FAST DIET
MEALS FOR ONE
Light Bite Recipes Under 100 Calories

Light Bacon & Eggs

Serves: 1 Calories: 94

Ingredients:

3 egg whites

1 slice lean back bacon

Low cal cooking spray

Salt & pepper to taste

1 tbsp freshly chopped chives

Method:

In a frying pan heat a little low cal cooking spray. Fry the bacon for 3 minutes. Break and separate the egg whites into a cup. Season and add to the frying pan beside the bacon. Keep on moving the eggs to scramble them. After 2-3 minutes the eggs and bacon should be ready. Tip onto a plate and serve with chopped chives over the top.

Mushroom Egg White Omelette

Serves: 1 Calories: 88

Ingredients:

3 egg whites

50g/2oz mushrooms

Salt & pepper to taste

1 tbsp chopped flat leaf parsley

1 slice (about 10g) low fat cheddar cheese, chopped

Method:

Gently sauté the mushrooms in a small frying pan with a little low cal cooking spray for a few minutes. Break and separate the egg whites into a bowl, season well and then tip the softened mushrooms, parsley and cheese into the egg whites. Add a little more low cal spray to the frying pan and pour in the egg and mushroom mixture. Cook until golden brown on the underside. Flip the omelette, cook for a minute or two more and serve.

Tuna Salad

Serves: 1 Calories: 90

Ingredients:

40g/1½oz tinned tuna steak in water

1 tsp low fat mayonnaise

1 gherkin, chopped

½ head romaine lettuce, shredded

Salt & pepper to taste

Method:

Flake the tuna and mix with the mayonnaise, chopped gherkin and seasoning. Sit on the shredded lettuce and serve.

Cucumber Cakes

Serves: 1 Calories: 97

Ingredients:

½ cucumber

1 tbsp low fat crème fraiche

1 tbsp low fat houmous

1 tbsp chopped dill

Method:

Cut the cucumber into 4 thick slices. Mix the crème fraiche and houmous together and spread equally over the top of each cucumber slice. Sprinkle the dill over the top and serve.

Thai Carrot Noodles

Serves: 1 Calories: 91

Ingredients:

1 tbsp fish sauce

1 tbsp lime juice

½ tsp brown sugar

1 shallot, finely chopped

½ red chilli, deseeded and finely chopped

1 carrot, cut into fine matchsticks

1 tbsp freshly chopped mint

50g/2oz Shirataki 'miracle' noodles

Method:

Cook the noodles as per the manufacturers instructions. Mix together the fish sauce, lime juice, sugar, shallots, chillies and carrots. Add to the noodles and sprinkle with chopped mint.

Balsamic Aubergine & Rocket Salad

Serves: 1 Calories: 96

Ingredients:

½ aubergine/egg plant, cut into small chunks

1 tbsp balsamic vinegar

50g/2oz rocket

Salt & pepper to taste

Low cal cooking spray

Method:

Pre-heat oven to 180C/350F/Gas 4. Spray the aubergine with low cal cooking oil. Season and spoon over the balsamic vinegar. Place on a baking tray and roast for 20-30 mins until soft and browned. Mix with the rocket and serve.

Lime Courgette Snack

Serves: 1 Calories: 94

Ingredients:

1 courgette/zucchini, sliced

½ red chilli, deseeded and finely chopped

50g/2oz spinach

1 tbsp lime juice

Low cal cooking oil

Method:

Heat a little low cal cooking spray in a frying pan and cook the courgette slices. Season well, add the chilli, spinach and lemon juice; cook for a minute longer until the spinach wilts and serve.

Cauliflower & Capers

Serves: 1 Calories: 95

Ingredients:

¼ head large cauliflower

½ carrot, grated

½ red onion, finely chopped

1 tsp capers, chopped

1 tbsp chopped parsley

2 tsp white wine vinegar

½ tsp Dijon mustard

1 tsp low fat mayonnaise

1 tbsp warm water

Method:

Split the cauliflower into little florets so that none are bigger than 2cm/1inch. Add to the carrots, red onion, capers and chopped parsley. Mix together the white wine vinegar, water, Dijon mustard and mayonnaise. Season well and toss through the cauliflower salad.

Rosemary Olives

Serves: 1 Calories: 92

Ingredients:

50g/2oz green olives

½ tsp chopped fresh rosemary

1 sundried tomato, finely chopped

½ tsp olive oil

Pinch of crushed sea salt

1 garlic clove, finely chopped

Method:

Toss all the ingredients together and chill.

Chilli Asparagus

Serves: 1 Calories: 98

Ingredients:

10 Asparagus spears

½ red chilli finely chopped

Low cal cooking spray

1 tsp balsamic vinegar

Method:

Trim the thick woody ends from the asparagus spears.
Cook the asparagus in salted boiling water for 2-3
minutes. Drain and rinse in cold water. Dry and set to one
side. Cover the spears with a little low cal cooking spray
and place in a hot frying pan. Cook for 3 minutes to brown
the spears, season and then add the chilli and balsamic
vinegar to the pan for a minute longer. Mix well and
serve.

Melon Fruit Cup

Serves: 1 Calories: 89

Ingredients:

¼ melon flesh, cubed

2 tbsp orange juice

Pinch brown sugar

40g/1 ½ oz raspberries

Method:

Gently combine all the ingredients together and serve in a cup.

Minted Grapefruit

Serves: 1 Calories: 95

Ingredients:

1 pink grapefruit

2 shallots, finely sliced

Pinch soft brown sugar

1 tbsp freshly chopped mint

1 tbsp freshly chopped coriander/cilantro

Low cal cooking spray

Method:

Peel and cut the grapefruit into slices. Gently sauté the chopped shallots in a little low cal cooking spray for a minute or two with a pinch of sugar. Arrange the grapefruit slices on a plate and scatter over the shallots and chopped herbs.

Cauliflower Cheese

Serves: 1 Calories: 94

Ingredients:

200g/7oz cauliflower florets

25g/1oz grated low fat cheddar cheese

Pinch of nutmeg

Salt & pepper to taste

Method:

Preheat oven to 325°F/160°C/gas 3

Break the cauliflower head into small florets and wash under a cold tap. Place in a small ovenproof dish, season and grate the cheese over the top. Add a pinch of nutmeg and bake for 20-30 mins or until the cauliflower is tender.

Lemon Sole

Serves: 1 Calories: 99

Ingredients:

100g/3½oz lemon sole fillet

2 tbsp lemon juice

2 spring onions/scallions finely chopped

Low cal cooking spray

Salt & pepper to taste

Method:

Preheat oven to 375°F/190°C/gas mark 5.

Place the sole in a shallow roasting tray with a little low cal spray. Coat in lemon juice, season and sprinkle the finely chopped spring onion over the top. Bake for 15 mins or until the fish is cooked through.

Tiger Prawns

Serves: 1 Calories: 94

Ingredients:

75g/3oz raw tiger prawns

1 tbsp low-fat mayonnaise

1 tsp lemon juice

Salt & pepper to taste

Method:

Combine the lemon juice with mayonnaise, season and set to one side. Heat a wok or frying pan until hot with a little low cal spray. Add the prawns, season and cook for approx. 5 mins or until prawns turn pink and are cooked through. Serve with the mayonnaise dip.

Spicy Watermelon Salad

Serves: 1 Calories: 60

Ingredients:

1 slice watermelon

1 small red chilli, deseeded and finely chopped

1 tsp freshly chopped coriander/cilantro

¼ red onion, finely chopped

1 tsp lime juice

Method:

Cube the watermelon and combine with chilli,
coriander/cilantro and lime juice for a sweet crunchy
snack with a kick.

White Bean Salad

Serves: 1 Calories: 94

Ingredients:

75g/3oz tinned cannellini beans

1 tbsp spring onions/scallions chopped

1 medium tomato, chopped

1 tsp lemon juice

Salt & pepper to taste

1 tbsp fresh chopped flat leaf parsley

Method:

Drain the beans and combine in a bowl with the spring onions, parsley, tomato and lemon juice. Season well and serve.

Raw Asparagus & Mushroom Salad

Serves: 1 Calories: 99

Ingredients:

6 asparagus spears

40g/1 ½ oz mushrooms, sliced

1 tsp fresh chopped flat leaf parsley

1 tsp lemon juice

½ tsp Parmesan cheese, grated

½ tsp olive oil

Salt & pepper to taste

Method:

Wash and remove any tough stalks from the asparagus and discard. Thinly slice the tender stalks. Wash the mushrooms and again thinly slice. Season and combine all ingredients in a bowl topped with grated Parmesan.

Skinny
5:2 FAST DIET
MEALS FOR ONE
50 Snacks Under 100 Calories

Inevitably there will be times throughout your fast days when hunger pangs may hit. Here's a list of useful 'grab & go' snack ideas to keep you on track.

Chocolate Banana: 100 calories
Half a frozen banana dipped in 2 squares of melted dark chocolate.

Frozen Grapes: 86 calories
125g/4oz of green or black grapes frozen.

Blueberry Yoghurt: 91 calories
100g/3½oz blueberries mixed with 2 tbsp of fat free Greek yoghurt.

Chocolate Strawberries: 72 calories
5 medium strawberries dipped in 2 squares of melted dark chocolate.

Spiced Apple: 95 calories
1 medium apple, cored & sliced; sprinkled with ½ tsp brown sugar and 1 tsp cinnamon. Bake in the oven until soft.

Latte: 93 calories
250ml/1 cup skimmed milk with 1 shot of espresso coffee.

Houmous & Veg Dips: 71 calories
2 tbsp low fat houmous with 1 carrot & 1 stalk celery cut into crudités.

Pistachios: 85 calories
1 small cup (around 25 nuts).

Beef Jerky: 40 calories
2 strips (4 inches) of smoked beef jerky.

Sweet Potato Fries: 95 calories
1 small sweet potato, peeled and sliced into thin matchsticks tossed in a little low cal cooking spray and cooked in the oven at
375F/190C/gas mark 5 for 10 mins turning twice.

Olives: 50 calories

6 Kalamata olives.

Asparagus & Boiled Egg: 98 calories

1 free range egg cooked to perfection (place egg in a pan of cold water, bring to the boil and simmer for exactly 3 minutes).

2 asparagus tips for dipping - steam the asparagus for 3-5 minutes.

Carrot & Raisin Salad: 100 calories

1 cup of shaved carrot mixed with 25g/1oz raisins and a splash of balsamic vinegar.

Baked Beans In Tomato Sauce: 70 calories

Choose the low salg and sugar canned options and measure 100g.

Smoked Salmon & Cream Cheese: 70 calories

28g/1oz wild smoked salmon with 1 tbsp low fat cream cheese.

Grapefruit: 45 calories

1/2 large pink grapefruit with 1 tsp sugar.

Melon & Parma Ham: 94 calories

1/16 wedge of watermelon with 2 slices of parma ham.

Popcorn: 97 calories

2 cups of air popped corn. Add 1 tsp of sugar.

Popcorn Cheese: 94 calories

2 cups of air popped corn. Add 1 tsp of grated parmesan cheese and a pinch of salt.

Grilled Sweet Peppers: 82 calories

1/2 each of green, red and yellow sweet peppers. Slice into 1 inch strip, mix in a bowl with 1 tbsp balsamic vinegar and place under a medium grill until tender.

Wasabi Peas: 68 calories

3 tbsp wasabi peas.

Pumpkin Seeds: 100 calories

2 tbsps of pumpkin seeds

Edamame Beans: 100 calories

1/4 cup of steamed edamame beans (4 mins) with a pinch of crushed sea salt.

Hardboiled egg: 78 calories

Place 1 medium free range egg in a pan of cold water and bring to the boil. Continue to simmer for 5 mins then allow to cool.

Frozen Banana: 90 calories

Peel and place in the freezer for 2 hours.

Pickled Gherkins: 50 calories

300g/12oz pickled gherkins.

Toast & Marmite: 100 calories

1 slice of wholemeal toast, low fat spread and marmite spread thinly.

Portabella Mushroom & Feta: 100 calories

1 medium portabella mushroom cap with 1 tsp low fat feta cheese. Fill the mushroom cap with feta, season and gently grill for 10 mins.

Cottage Cheese & Celery: 75 calories

75g/3oz low fat natural cottage cheese with 3 celery sticks.

Chicken Drumstick: 89 calories

1 small skinless chicken drumstick, ¼ tsp of dried mixed herbs, low cal spray. Sprinkle the drumstick with the herbs and give a couple of sprays of low cal cooking spray. Cook in a preheated oven at 375F/190C/gas mark 5 for 20 mins or until cooked through.

Guacamole & Chips: 96 calories

1 tbsp of low fat guacamole with 8 tortilla chips.

Bagel & Smoked Salmon: 100 calories

½ mini wholegrain bagel with one slice of smoked salmon, lemon juice and cracked pepper.

Crackers & Peanut Butter: 93 calories

2 crackers/crackerbread thinly spread with peanut butter.

Strawberries & Goat's Cheese: 98 calories
10 strawberries dipped in 2 tsp low fat goat's cheese.

Cherries & Fromage Frais: 97 calories
60ml/ ¼ cup low fat fromage frais + 5 cherries.

Cinnamon Orange: 80 calories
1 medium orange, peeled and split into segments. In a bowl mix together 1 tsp of lemon juice, 1 tsp orange juice and a pinch of cinnamon. Pour over orange segments and serve.

Paprika Eggs: 100 calories
I medium hard boiled egg, sliced. Cover the egg in 1 tsp olive oil and spindle with paprika.

Cottage Cheese Salad: 95 calories
50g/2oz low-fat natural cottage cheese topped with 3 chopped spring onions/scallions. Chop ½ red pepper, mix and serve.

Tricolore: 94 calories
1 slice of low fat mozzarella cheese, 3 cherry tomatoes and 3 fresh basil leaves, Salt & pepper to serve.

Cottage Cheese & Pineapple: 72 calories
50g low fat cottage cheese with 50g fresh pineapple.

Black-eyed Beans: 90 calories
50g/2oz tinned beans, 1 medium chopped tomato, 1 tbsp chopped onion and 1/2 tsp minced garlic, combine. Season and serve.

Warm Goat's Cheese with Sugar Snap Peas
100g/3 ½ oz sugar snap peas steamed for 4 minutes. Warm 20g/ ¾ oz goat's cheese for 10 secs in a microwave.

Tuna & Capers: 79 calories
75g/3oz tinned tuna mixed with 1 tbsp capers and 1 tsp lemon juice.

Celery & Cream Cheese; 68 calories
3 celery stalks with 2 tsp low-fat cream cheese.

Honey Yoghurt: 79 calories

120ml/ ½ cup fat free Greek yoghurt with 1 tsp runny honey.

Cheesy tomatoes: 89 calories

2 plum tomatoes split in half, topped with 1 tbsp breadcrumbs and 1 tbsp parmesan cheese. Bake in a hot oven for 45-60 mins.

Marinated Smoked Salmon: 97 calories

50g/2oz smoked salmon, 3 radishes finely sliced, 3 spring onions/scallions chopped. Marinate all ingredients win ½ tbsp fresh orange juice + ½ tbsp red wine vinegar for 10 mins then serve.

Curried Tuna: 95 calories

75g/3 oz tinned tuna mixed with 1 tsp mild curry powder and 1 tbsp chopped red onion.

Apple Cider Cucumber salad: 42 calories

100g/3 ½ oz diced cucumber mixed with 2 tbsp chopped red onion and 1 tbsp cider vinegar.

Chickpea, Lemon & Spring Onions: 78 calories

50g/2oz tinned chickpeas, 1 tbsp lemon juice, 3 chopped spring onions/scallions. Combine all ingredients and serve.

Curried Sweet Potato: 90 calories

100g/3 ½ oz diced sweet potato, 1 tsp curry powder. Cook the sweet potato for 6 mins in a microwave then mash with curry powder and salt & pepper to taste.

Skinny
5:2 FAST DIET
MEALS FOR ONE
Recipes Under 200 Calories

Vegetable Chilli

Serves: 1 Calories: 170

Ingredients:

1 garlic clove, crushed

1 red chilli, deseeded and finely chopped

½ tsp ground cumin

½ tsp ground coriander

75g/3oz fresh mushrooms, sliced

100g/3½oz chopped tomatoes (tinned or fresh)

100g/3½oz tinned kidney beans

75g/3oz green beans, chopped

1 tbsp low fat crème fraiche

1 tsp chopped chives

Salt & pepper to taste

Low cal cooking spray

Method:

Gently sauté the garlic and chilli in a little low cal spray for a couple of minutes. Add the cumin, coriander, mushrooms, tomatoes, kidney beans, green beans and 2 tbsp water. Stir well, season and leave to simmer for 10-15 minutes or until all the veg is tender and the chilli is nice and thick. If you prefer more of a crunch add the green beans later in the cooking. Dollop the crème fraiche into the middle of the chilli and serve with the chives sprinkled over the top.

Japanese Aubergine

Serves: 1 Calories: 194

Ingredients:

1 aubergine/egg plant

½ tsp golden caster sugar

1 tsp lemon juice

2 spring onions/scallions, cut into fine lengths

1 tbsp miso paste

1 tbsp sake

50g/2oz rocket

Salt & pepper to taste

1 lime wedge

Low cal cooking spray

Method:

Pre-heat the oven to 180C/350F/gas 4.

Cut the aubergine/eggplant in half lengthways. Brush the exposed flesh with a little low cal cooking spray and season well. Place on a baking tray and cook for 15-25 minutes or until the flesh is tender and remove from the oven.

Heat the grill up and mix together the sake, miso, sugar & lemon juice and brush it all onto the roasted aubergine flesh. Place under the hot grill and cook for 2 minutes or until the flesh turns golden. Serve with the rocket, spring onions and a wedge of lime.

Super Simple Squash Curry Snack

Serves: 1 Calories: 179

Ingredients:

½ onion, sliced

2 tsp curry paste

125g/4oz butternut squash, peeled and cubed

1 tomato, quartered

50g/2oz spinach, chopped

60ml/¼ cup water

1 tsp chopped coriander/cilantro

Salt & pepper to taste

Low cal cooking spray

Method:

Gently sauté the onion in a little low cal spray for a few minutes. Add the curry paste and cook for a further minute before adding the squash, tomatoes and water. Season, stir well, cover and leave to simmer for 10-15 minutes or until the squash is tender. Add the spinach and warm through for a minute. Serve with the chopped coriander sprinkled over the top.

Tomato & Basil Spaghetti

Serves: 1 Calories: 191

Ingredients:

50g/2oz spaghetti

1 garlic clove, crushed

100g/3 ½ oz tinned chopped tomatoes

½ vegetable stock cube

1 tsp tomato purée/paste

½ tsp sugar

1 tsp dried basil

1 tsp fresh chopped basil

Low cal cooking spray

Method:

Cook the spaghetti in boiling salted water until tender.
Meanwhile gently sauté the garlic in a little low cal
cooking spray for 1 minute. Crumble the stock cube and
add it to the garlic along with the chopped tomatoes,
tomato puree, sugar and dried basil; simmer for a few
minutes. When the spaghetti is cooked, drain and place
into the tomato pan. Combine well. Sprinkle with the fresh
basil and serve.

Fried Zucchini & Eggs

Serves: 1 Calories: 197

Ingredients:

200g/7oz courgettes/zucchini, chopped

100g/3½oz cherry tomatoes

1 garlic clove, crushed

1 free range egg

1 tbsp chopped fresh basil

Salt & pepper to taste

Low cal cooking spray

Method:

Cut the tomatoes in half and gently sauté along with the courgettes and garlic in a little low cal spray for 5 minutes. Break the egg into the pan, season, cover and leave to cook for 2-4 minutes or until the egg is cooked. Serve with the fresh basil sprinkled over.

Smoked Salmon & Poppy Seeds

Serves: 1 Calories: 196

Ingredients:

1 tsp poppy seeds, lightly toasted

1 orange

1 tsp red wine vinegar

½ tsp sesame oil

100g/3½oz smoked salmon

5 radishes, trimmed and finely sliced

1 spring onion/scallion, finely sliced lengthways

Salt & pepper to taste

Method:

First, grate the zest of the orange and then squeeze out the juice. Mix both these ingredients together with the poppy seeds, red wine vinegar and sesame oil. Add the salmon slices, radishes and spring onions and combine gently. Season and arrange on a plate making sure the salmon slices are spread out. Serve immediately.

Ginger Curry Prawns

Serves: 1 Calories: 168

Ingredients:

100g/3 ½ oz raw fresh peeled prawns

1 tbsp fat free Greek yogurt

½ onion, chopped

½ tsp turmeric

½ tsp cumin

½ tsp ground ginger

Pinch dried chilli flakes

1 garlic clove, crushed

100g/3½oz tinned chopped tomatoes

1 tsp chopped fresh coriander/cilantro

Salt & pepper to taste

Low cal cooking spray

Method:

Gently sauté the onion in a little low cal cooking spray for a few minutes. Add all the other ingredients, except the yoghurt, and leave to simmer for 10 minutes or until the prawns are cooked through. Remove from the heat and stir in the yoghurt. Season and serve sprinkled with the fresh coriander.

Paprika Prawn Cocktail

Serves: 1 Calories: 194

Ingredients:

75g/3oz raw fresh peeled prawns

1 garlic clove, crushed

½ tsp paprika

½ tsp chilli powder

1 tomato, chopped

½ tsp runny honey

1 tsp fresh chopped coriander/cilantro

½ head romaine lettuce, shredded

¼ small ripe avocado, cubed

1 wedge fresh lemon

Low cal cooking spray

Method:

Gently sauté the prawns and garlic in a little low cal coking spray. Add the paprika and chilli; cook for a few minutes until the prawns turn pink and are cooked through. Stir in the honey and leave to cool.

Meanwhile, arrange the shredded lettuce, chopped tomatoes and avocado into a large wine glass. Place the cooled prawns on top and serve with the lemon wedge.

Prawn Mayo Open Sandwich

Serves: 1 Calories: 184

Ingredients:

1 tomato, sliced

Handful of lettuce leaves

1 slice wholemeal bread

1 tsp low fat mayonnaise

1 tsp ketchup

1 tsp fresh chopped dill

1 tsp lemon juice

75g/3oz cooked, peeled prawns

¼ cucumber, sliced

Method:

Mix together the mayonnaise, ketchup and lemon juice. Add the prawns, tomato, cucumber and lettuce leaves. Season and serve on top of the wholemeal bread with the chopped dill sprinkled over.

Beef Stir-Fry Snack

Serves: 1 Calories: 194

Ingredients:

100g/3½oz lean sirloin steak

½ red chilli, deseeded and chopped

1 tsp oyster sauce

50g/2oz mixed salad leaves

2 tsp chopped basil leaves

Salt & pepper to taste

Low cal cooking spray

Method:

Slice the steak very thinly and season.

Spray a little low cal cooking oil into a frying pan and bring to a high heat. Add the steak strips and chopped chilli and stir-fry for about 2 minutes. Add the oyster sauce and continue to cook until the meat is coated. Take off the heat and toss through the basil. Serve immediately on a bed of salad leaves.

Seared Beef & Rocket

Serves: 1 Calories: 189

Ingredients:

100g/3½oz fillet steak

2 shallots, sliced

1 tbsp lemon juice

50g/2oz rocket

Salt & pepper to taste

Low cal cooking spray

Method:

Season the steak and coat with a little low cal spray. Put a dry frying pan on a high heat and cook on each side for 2 minutes. Put the steak to one side and pour the lemon juice into the pan to combine with the meat juices. Take off the heat and stir the shallots through the lemon juice.

Thinly slice the steak, season and sit on top of the rocket. Tip the lemony shallots over the top.

Sweet Asian Steak Snack

Serves: 1 Calories: 191

Ingredients:

2 tsp soy sauce

1 tsp balsamic vinegar

½ tsp honey

75g/3oz lean rump steak

½ carrot

½ fennel bulb

½ red onion

1 tbsp lime juice

1 tbsp chopped coriander

Salt & pepper to taste

Method:

Mix together the soy sauce, balsamic vinegar and honey. Brush the mixture onto the steak and leave to marinate. Meanwhile, grate the carrot and slice the fennel & red onion. Toss with the chopped coriander and put to one side on a plate.

Put a dry frying pan on a high heat and add the steak. Cook for 2 minutes each side. Rest for a further 2 minutes and slice very thinly. Season and serve the steak on top of the fennel salad.

Thai Chicken Curry Snack

Serves: 1 Calories: 193

Ingredients:

60ml/ ¼ cup low fat coconut milk

75g/3oz chicken breast, cubed

2 cherry tomatoes, chopped

1 tsp Thai red curry paste

25g/1oz green beans, chopped

25g/1oz baby corn, chopped

Salt & pepper to taste

1 tsp chopped coriander/cilantro

Low cal cooking spray

Method:

Season the chicken and use a little low cal spray to cook in a small frying pan. Cook for 4-6 minutes or until the chicken is cooked through. Add the curry paste and stir well. Reduce the heat and add the coconut milk and vegetables. Cover and leave to gently simmer for 5 minutes. By this time the milk and vegetables will be warmed through, still firm but not over cooked. Serve scattered with the chopped coriander.

Tamarind Chicken With Tomato & Onion Salad

Serves: 1 Calories: 197

Ingredients:

75g/3oz chicken breasts, cubed

2 tsp tamarind paste

½ tsp ground ginger

½ tsp chilli powder

½ tsp caster sugar

75g/3oz fresh tomatoes, sliced

½ red onion, sliced

1 tsp fresh chopped mint leaves

1 lemon wedge

Salt & pepper to taste

Method:

Pre-heat the grill to medium. Add the cubed chicken to a bowl with the tamarind, ginger, sugar and chilli powder. Season and combine well. Place the chicken under the grill and cook for approx. 6-8 minutes or until the chicken is cooked through. Arrange the sliced tomatoes and onion on a plate and put the cooked chicken on the side. Season, sprinkle with the chopped mint and serve with a lemon wedge to squeeze over the top.

Chicken Satay Snack

Serves: 1 Calories: 157

Ingredients:

75g/3oz chicken breast

2 tsp smooth peanut butter

1 tbsp soy sauce

1 tsp water

½ baby gem lettuce

1 tsp flat leaf parsley to serve

Method:

Pre-heat the grill to medium. Combine the peanut butter, water and soy in a bowl. Cube your chicken breast and add to the bowl, stirring to coat each piece of chicken with a thin layer of soy-peanut butter.

Place your chicken pieces under the grill and cook for about 6-8 minutes or until the chicken is cooked through. Serve with lettuce and parsley.

Lemon & Thyme Chicken

Serves: 1 Calories: 196

Ingredients:

100g/3½oz chicken breast

½ lemon cut into slices

1 tsp dried thyme

2 tsp runny honey

50g/2oz bean sprouts

1 sprig of bashed rosemary

Salt & pepper to taste

Low cal cooking spray

Method:

Preheat the grill to med/high. Place the chicken breast in a small, shallow dish with a little low cal cooking spray. Season and cook for 5 minutes. Mix together the thyme, rosemary & honey; brush onto the chicken. Place the lemon slices on top and continue to cook for a further 8-10 minutes or until the chicken is cooked through. Remove from the heat and slice the chicken. Meanwhile, add the raw bean sprouts to the hot baking dish and mix to coat in the juices. Serve with the chicken slices.

Zingy Chicken Salad

Serves: 1 Calories: 194

Ingredients:

75g/3oz cooked chicken breast, shredded

1 tsp caster sugar

50g/2oz mixed salad leaves

1 tbsp chopped fresh coriander/cilantro

¼ red onion, thinly sliced

½ chilli, deseeded and thinly sliced

¼ cucumber, halved lengthways, sliced

1 tbsp fish sauce

1 tbsp lime juice

Method:

Mix together the chopped chilli, fish sauce, lime juice and sugar. Place the salad leaves, cucumber and onion in a bowl. Add the shredded chicken and toss with the fish sauce dressing. When properly combined sprinkle with chopped coriander/cilantro and serve.

Sweet Pork & Spinach Snack

Serves: 1 Calories: 199

Ingredients:

100g/3½oz pork tenderloin fillet

1 tbsp soy sauce

1 tsp honey

1 tbsp fresh orange juice

½ tsp ground ginger

50g/2oz spinach

Method:

Pre-heat the oven to 200C/fan 180C/gas 6.

Combine the soy sauce, honey, orange juice and ginger together. Coat the pork fillet with this marinade. Place in a shallow ovenproof dish and roast for approx. 20 minutes or until the pork is cooked through. Remove from the heat and slice thinly. Meanwhile, plunge the spinach into salted boiling water and simmer for 1 minute. Drain and serve with the sliced pork.

Clear Pork Snack Bowl

Serves: 1 Calories: 196

Ingredients:

100g/3½oz pork tenderloin

250ml/1 cup chicken stock/broth

1 tsp soy sauce

½ tsp Chinese five-spice powder

½ tsp ground ginger

Pinch chilli flakes

½ pak choi, shredded

2 spring onions/scallions, sliced lengthways

Salt & pepper to taste

Method:

First prepare the pork by slicing into strips, seasoning and brushing with Chinese five-spice powder. Place the pork, chicken stock, soy sauce, ginger, chilli flakes and pak choi into a pan. Gently simmer for approx. 6-8 minutes, or until the pork is cooked through. Take off the heat and tip into a bowl. Season and serve with the spring onion lengths sprinkled over the top.

Pork Pot Noodle Snack

Serves: 1 Calories: 191

Ingredients:

25g/1oz thick rice noodles
50g/2oz beansprouts
1 tbsp lime juice
1 tsp each fish sauce & soy sauce
Pinch brown sugar
½ red onion, sliced
1 baby gem lettuce, shredded
½ tsp each ground ginger & paprika
75g/3oz lean pork mince
Salt & pepper to taste
Low cal cooking spray

Method:

Mix together the lime, soy, sugar and fish sauce.

Plunge the noodles and beansprouts into salted boiling water and leave to cook for a few minutes. When the noodles are tender, drain and combine with the fish sauce mix.

Meanwhile, fry the mince in a little low cal cooking spray. Add the ginger and paprika and stir-fry for 6-8 minutes or until cooked through. Season and add the noodle and beansprouts to the pan. Combine well and serve with shredded lettuce.

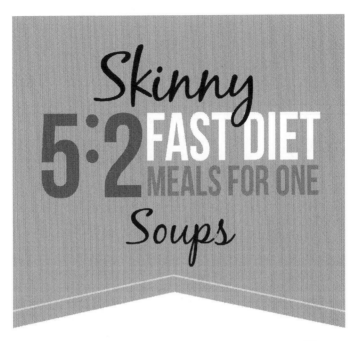

Soups are a great, filling, wholesome meal choice. These recipes are all individual portions, but more often than not it makes sense to prepare larger batches of soup and save in single servings for another time. If you do decide you want make multiple servings just increase the quantities evenly across the ingredients.

Soups can also be 'filled' out by adding a little more stock or skimmed milk to give additional quantity with very little added calories.

Soups make a great warming lunch when you are at work and can easily be made in advance to heat up when you need it

Try having one of the lower calorie soups as a snack in a thermo-mug to sip on while you are travelling or watching TV

Tuscan Bean Soup

Serves: 1 Calories: 179

Ingredients:

½ onion, chopped
1 garlic clove, crushed
1 stick celery, chopped
1 courgette/zucchini, chopped
100g/3½oz chopped tomatoes (tinned or fresh)
250ml/1 cup vegetable stock/broth
100g/ 3½oz tinned mixed beans
 ½ tsp dried oregano
½ tsp dried basil
1 tbsp tomato puree/paste
1 tsp flat leaf parsley, chopped
Salt & pepper to taste

Method:

Place everything in a saucepan, except the parsley, beans
& courgette. Simmer for 10 minutes. Add the chopped
beans and courgettes and heat through for another 5
minutes or until all the vegetables are tender and cooked
through. Season and serve with the chopped parsley
sprinkled on top.

Chicken, Leek & Prune Soup

Serves: 1 Calories: 188

Ingredients:

75g/3oz chicken breast, cooked

½ leek, chopped

4 pitted prunes, chopped

250ml/1 cup chicken stock/broth

½ tsp dried thyme

½ tsp dried rosemary

Salt & pepper to taste

Low cal cooking spray

Method:

Shred the cooked chicken breast. Gently sauté the leeks in a little low cal spray in a saucepan for a few minutes. Add the herbs and chicken and season. Add the stock and bring to the boil. Cover and leave to simmer for 20 minutes. Add the prunes and warm through for a further 5 minutes. Make sure everything is tender and piping hot. Adjust seasoning and serve. You can pulse the soup in a blender if you prefer a smoother consistency.

Beef & Barley Soup

Serves: 1 Calories: 191

Ingredients:

15g/½oz pearl barley (soaked in water overnight)

310ml/ 1¼ cups beef stock/broth

½ tsp dried oregano

½ tsp dried parsley

50g/2oz lean sirloin steak, very finely sliced

½ carrot, chopped

½ leek, chopped

1 tsp fresh basil, chopped

Salt & pepper to taste

Method:

Combine the soaked barley, stock and dried herbs in a saucepan and bring to the boil. Add all the other ingredients, except the fresh basil, to the pan and season. Cover and leave to simmer gently for 40 minutes or until the barley and beef are tender. Adjust the seasoning and serve with the basil sprinkled over the top.

Red Pepper & Yoghurt Soup

Serves: 1 Calories: 111

Ingredients:

1 red pepper, chopped

½ onion, chopped

½ red chilli, deseeded and chopped

120ml/½ cup tomato passatta/sieved tomatoes

120ml/ ½ cup vegetable broth/stock

1 tsp dried basil

1 tsp chopped fresh dill

Salt & pepper to taste

1 tbsp fat free Greek yoghurt

Method:

Bring all the ingredients, except the chopped basil and yoghurt, to the boil in a saucepan. Cover and leave to simmer for 20 minutes. When the vegetables are tender use a blender or food processor to blend the soup into a smooth consistency. Adjust the seasoning and serve with the yoghurt gently dolloped into the centre of the bowl and the fresh dill sprinkled on top.

Beetroot Soup

Serves: 1 Calories: 149

Ingredients:

½ onion chopped

75g/3oz potato, chopped

½ small cooking apple, peeled, cored and chopped

1 tbsp water

½ tsp dried cumin

½ tsp dried coriander/cilantro

125g/4oz fresh cooked beetroot, diced

½ tsp lemon juice

250ml/1 cup veg stock/broth

1 tbsp low fat crème fraiche

Salt & pepper to taste

Method:

Add all the ingredients, except the crème fraiche and lemon, into a saucepan and bring to the boil. Cover and leave to simmer for 20 minutes. When the vegetables are tender use a blender, or food processor, to blend the soup into a smooth consistency. Stir through the lemon juice and adjust the seasoning. Serve with the crème fraiche gently swirled through.

Spicy Apricot & Apple Soup

Serves: 1 Calories: 182

Ingredients:

40g/1½oz dried apricots, (soaked in water over night and chopped)

1 apple, cored, peeled & chopped

½ onion, chopped

1 tsp lime juice

250ml/1 cup vegetable stock/broth

Pinch of nutmeg & cinnamon

½ tsp dried cumin

¼ tsp chilli powder (optional)

1 tbsp fat free Greek yoghurt

Salt & Pepper to taste

Method:

Add all the ingredients, except the yoghurt and lime juice, into a saucepan and bring to the boil. Cover and leave to simmer for 20 minutes. When the vegetables are tender, use a blender or food processor to blend the soup into a smooth consistency. Stir through the lime juice and adjust the seasoning. Serve with the yoghurt dolloped on top.

Coconut & Crab Soup

Serves: 1 Calories: 181

Ingredients:

2 tsp Thai red curry paste

½ red pepper/bell pepper sliced

60ml/ ¼ cup low fat coconut milk

120ml/ ½ cup fish stock/broth

2 tsp fish sauce

100g/3½oz white crab meat (fresh or tinned)

1 tsp chopped coriander/cilantro

Salt & pepper to taste

Low cal cooking spray

Method:

Gently sauté the sliced pepper in a little low cal spray. When the pepper softens add the curry paste and stir through. Add the stock, fish sauce & crab meat and gently cook for a few minutes. Season and gently stir in the coconut milk. Warm through for a few minutes. Adjust the seasoning and serve with the chopped coriander sprinkled over the top.

Anchovy Rice Soup

Serves: 1 Calories: 155

Ingredients:

75g/3oz white crab meat (fresh or tinned)

1 tbsp long grain rice

120ml/ ½ cup skimmed milk

120ml/ ½ cup fish stock/broth

1 tsp anchovy paste

1 tsp lemon juice

1 tsp chopped flat leaf parsley

1 tbsp fat free Greek yoghurt

Salt & pepper to taste

Method:

Gently bring the rice and milk to the boil in a pan. Cover and simmer for approx. 10 minutes or until the rice is tender. Add half the crab meat along with the fish stock & anchovy paste then warm through. Use a blender or food processor to blend the soup into a smooth consistency. Return to the pan and add the rest of the crab meat for a minute or two. Take off the heat, add the yoghurt and lemon juice and stir through. Adjust the seasoning and sprinkle with flat leaf parsley.

Spiced Pea Soup

Serves: 1 Calories: 198

Ingredients:

½ onion, chopped

50g/2oz potatoes, peeled & chopped

1 clove garlic, crushed

½ tsp ground coriander

½ tsp ground cumin

½ tsp ground ginger

250ml/1 cup vegetable stock/broth

75g/3oz frozen peas

1 tsp chopped fresh mint

60ml/ ¼ cup skimmed milk

1 tbsp fat free Greek yoghurt

Low cal cooking spray

Method:

Gently sauté the onions and potato in a little low cal spray until the onion begins to soften. Add the garlic and dried spices and stir for a minute or two. Add the stock and peas, cover and leave to simmer for 15 minutes or until the potatoes are tender. Use a blender or food processor to blend the soup into a smooth consistency. Return to the pan and add the milk. Warm through, take off the heat, add the yoghurt and stir through. Adjust the seasoning and sprinkle with the chopped mint.

Mushroom Noodle Soup

Serves: 1 Calories: 166

Ingredients:

50g/2oz fresh mushrooms, sliced

250ml/1 cup vegetable stock/broth

25g/1oz fine egg noodles

1 garlic clove, crushed

½ tsp ground ginger

1 tsp soy sauce

75g/3oz beansprouts

½ onion, chopped

1 tsp ketchup

1 tsp fresh coriander/cilantro, chopped

Salt & pepper to taste

Low cal cooking spray

Method:

Gently sauté the mushrooms, garlic and onion in a little low cal spray for a few minutes. When the onion softens add the ginger and stir through, cooking for a minute or two longer.

Place in a pan with the stock, noodles, soy sauce and ketchup. Season, cover and simmer for 5-10 minutes until the noodles are tender. Add the beansprouts and warm for a minute or two. Adjust the seasoning and serve with the chopped coriander sprinkled over the top.

Skinny
5:2 FAST DIET
MEALS FOR ONE
Smoothies Under 200 Calories

Smoothies

Smoothies are a fantastic way to supplement your 5:2 Diet fast days. A smoothie is basically a thick blended drink which in addition to fruit or vegetables usually includes crushed ice, yoghurt or milk (or milk alternative). Smoothies can be a fantastic source of vitamins and nutrients and they taste great. They help make up the essential daily intake of fruit (and veg) and unlike many of the store bought drinks, the following recipes contain no added sugar and all fall under 100 or 200 calories.

Tips For A Perfect Smoothie

Everyone has their own tips for how to make the perfect smoothie and indeed you should experiment and take advice from lots of different sources to find what works best for you. To start you off follow our top tips for whizzing up the best smoothies first time around.

Add your liquid first, not fruit, to prevent your blender blade becoming blunt or damaged.

Freeze your fruit. If you want to save time in preparation you can freeze your favourite fruits in advance. Pretty much all fruit is fine to freeze for smoothies. Plus you won't need to use as much ice when you blend.

Choose good quality, seasonal and if possible organic fruit. Seasonal fruit will have a much stronger flavour and organic fruit should be free from any chemicals or preservatives. Freezing keeps all the goodness locked inside.

Avoid adding too many sweeteners such as sugar, ice cream etc. Most fruits have natural sweetness in them. Use natural sweetener such as Agave syrup, honey or Maple syrup if you can.

Blender Advice

A blender is an essential piece of kit for making smoothies. Some use a blending attachment to their mixer or others a stand-alone appliance – both will do the job.

How smooth do you like your smoothie? If you prefer a super smooth consistency then perhaps a blender with more power may be better for you.

Speed – do you need multiple speeds on your blender? For most, one setting will do the job nicely but as before if you prefer a smoother consistency you may wish to consider multiple speed settings.

Cleaning - Your blender will need a good clean after each use. You will generally need to remove the blade to do this – some blenders are simpler to reassemble than others. If you use a dishwasher makes sure the blender parts are dishwasher safe. Another good tip is to use freshly squeezed lemon juice all over to help zap those stubborn marks.

Breakfast Smoothie

Serves: 1 Calories: 120

Ingredients:
75g/3oz blackberries
120ml/ ½ cup apple juice
½ banana
Handful of ice cubes

Method:
Combine all the ingredients into a blender and blend until smooth.

Raspberry & Almond Milk Smoothie

Serves: 1 Calories: 190

Ingredients:
60ml/ ¼ cup almond milk
50g/2oz raspberries
½ banana
1 tsp agave nectar
Handful of ice cubes

Method:
Combine all the ingredients into a blender and blend until smooth.

Cherry Hit Smoothie

Serves: 1 Calories: 193

Ingredients:
50g/2oz cherries
1 kiwi fruit
60 ml/¼ cup pure orange juice
60 ml/¼ cup coconut water
½ tsp agave nectar
Handful of ice

Method:
Combine all the ingredients into a blender and blend until smooth.

Peach, Apple & Cucumber Smoothie

Serves: 1 Calories: 143

Ingredients:
1 medium peach, peeled and stoned
60ml/ ¼ cup pure apple juice
¼ cucumber, peeled
2 tsp lime juice
1 tsp fresh mint, finely chopped
1 tsp agave nectar
2 handfuls of ice

Method:
Combine all the ingredients into a blender and blend until smooth.

Tropical Smoothie

Serves: 1 Calories: 169

Ingredients:
½ mango, peeled and stoned
½ banana
60ml/ ¼ cup fat free peach yoghurt
60ml/ ¼ cup cranberry juice
Handful Of ice
Method:
Combine all the ingredients into a blender and blend until smooth.

Blueberry Banana Smoothie

Serves: 1 Calories: 145

Ingredients:
50g/2oz blueberries
1 banana
120ml/ ½ cup pineapple juice
Handful of ice

Method:
Combine all the ingredients into a blender and blend until smooth.

Ginger & Strawberry Smoothie

Serves: 1 Calories: 195

Ingredients:
120ml/ ½ cup skimmed milk
1 banana
50g/2oz strawberries
1 tsp fresh ginger finely chopped
1 tsp agave nectar
Handful of ice
Method:
Combine all the ingredients into a blender and blend until smooth.

Pomegranate, Kiwi & Berry Smoothie

Serves: 1 Calories: 189

Ingredients:
½ banana
1 kiwi, peeled
50g/3oz blueberries
120ml/½ cup cranberry juice
Handful of ice

Method:
Combine all the ingredients into a blender and blend until smooth.

Peach & Ginger Smoothie

Serves: 1 Calories: 160

Ingredients:
2 medium peaches, skinned and stoned
120ml/½ cup unsweetened apple juice
½ tsp ground ginger
1 tsp agave nectar
Handful of ice

Method:
Combine all the ingredients into a blender and blend until smooth.

Strawberry Spinach Smoothie

Serves: 1 Calories: 157

Ingredients:
½ banana
50g/2oz strawberries
handful of fresh spinach leaves
60ml/ ¼ cup fat free vanilla yoghurt
1 tsp honey
Handful of ice

Method:
Combine all the ingredients into a blender and blend until smooth.

Cranberry & Apple Smoothie

Serves: 1 Calories: 120

Ingredients:
1 apple, cored and chopped
75g/3oz fresh cranberries
1 tsp honey
Handful of ice

Method:
Combine all the ingredients into a blender and blend until smooth.

Spiced Up Banana Smoothie

Serves: 1 Calories: 144

Ingredients:
1 banana
120ml/ ½ cup skimmed milk
¼ tsp ground cinnamon
¼ tsp ground nutmeg
¼ tsp ground cloves
Handful of ice

Method:
Combine all the ingredients into a blender and blend until smooth.

Rhubarb Smoothie

Serves: 1 Calories: 158

Ingredients:
2 precooked rhubarb stalks
60ml/ ¼ cup orange juice
60ml/ ¼ cup fat free plain yoghurt
1 tbsp agave nectar
Handful of ice

Method:
Combine all the ingredients into a blender and blend until smooth.

Green Veg Smoothie

Serves: 1 Calories: 128

Ingredients:
¼ head of broccoli
1 apple, peeled & cored
120ml/ ½ cup fat free yoghurt
1 tbsp lime juice
4 tbsp pineapple juice
Handful of ice

Method:
Bring a pan of water to the boil and add the broccoli florets. Cook for 5-6 mins or until tender.
Remove from the heat, drain and cool. Place the yoghurt, broccoli, cucumber, lime, pineapple juice and ice into blender and blend until smooth.

Spinach, Grape & Kiwi Smoothie

Serves: 1 Calories: 140

Ingredients:
75g/3oz green grapes
1 kiwi, peeled
Handful of spinach
120ml/ ½ cup watermelon juice
Handful of ice

Method:
Combine all the ingredients into a blender and blend until smooth.

Vanilla & Banana Smoothie

Serves: 1 Calories: 115

Ingredients:
½ banana
120ml/ ½ cup fat free vanilla yoghurt
Handful of ice

Method:
Combine all the ingredients into a blender and blend until smooth.

Coffee Smoothie

Serves: 1 Calories: 188

Ingredients:
1 tsp espresso powder1 banana
120ml/ ½ cup fat free plain yoghurt
50g/2oz strawberries
¼ tsp cinnamon
1 tsp cocoa powder

Method:
Combine all the ingredients into a blender and blend until smooth.

Strawberry & Banana Smoothie

Serves: 1 Calories: 140
Ingredients:
120ml/ ½ cup plain fat free yoghurt
½ banana
5 strawberries
Handful of ice

Method:
Combine all the ingredients into a blender and blend until smooth.

Mixed Berry Smoothie

Serves: 1 Calories: 150
Ingredients:
½ banana
75g/3oz mixed berries
120ml/ ½ cup plain fat free yoghurt
Handful of ice.

Method:
Combine all the ingredients into a blender and blend until smooth.

Kiwi & Strawberry Smoothie

Serves: 1 Calories: 170
Ingredients:
1 banana
1 kiwi fruit
5 strawberries
1 tsp agave nectar
60ml/1/2 cup skimmed milk
Handful of ice

Method:
Combine all the ingredients into a blender and blend until smooth.

Skinny
5:2 FAST DIET
MEALS FOR ONE
Recipes Under 300 Calories

Healthy Club Sandwich

Serves: 1 Calories: 270

Ingredients:

2 slices granary bread

handful of rocket

1 carrot

1 tsp lemon juice

2 tbsp low fat houmous

2 tomatoes, chopped

Salt & pepper to taste

Method:

Lightly toast the granary bread and spread the houmous over both slices. Grate the carrot and place in a bowl with the lemon juice, rocket and chopped tomatoes. Season well and load onto one of the houmous covered granary slices. Top with the other slice, cut in half and serve.

Chickpea & Pumpkin Curry

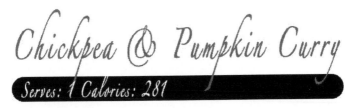

Serves: 1 Calories: 281

Ingredients:

2 tsp Thai yellow curry paste

200g/7oz pumpkin flesh, cubed

120ml/ ½ cup vegetable stock/broth

60ml/ ¼ cup low fat coconut milk

75g/3oz tinned chickpeas

½ onion, sliced

1 stalk lemongrass

1 tsp mustard seed

1 tbsp lime juice

1 tbsp fresh chopped coriander/cilantro

Salt & pepper to taste

Low cal cooking spray

Method:

Add a little low cal spray to a frying pan and gently sauté the onion and mustard seeds. Take the tip off the lemongrass stalk and bash the stalk with a rolling pin to release the flavour. Add the curry paste and lemongrass; cook for a few minutes. Add the pumpkin, chickpeas and stock; cover and leave to simmer for 8-10 minutes, or until the pumpkin is tender. Add the coconut milk and gently warm through. Serve with chopped coriander/cilantro sprinkled over the top.

Sun Blush Barley Salad

Serves: 1 Calories: 299

Ingredients:

200g/7oz butternut squash, cubed

40g/1½ oz pearl barley

100g/3½ oz purple sprouting broccoli, roughly chopped

25g/1oz sun blush tomatoes, finely sliced

5 black olives, chopped

50g/2oz watercress

1 tbsp each chopped fresh basil & balsamic vinegar

1 tsp each extra-virgin olive oil, Dijon mustard & capers

½ garlic clove crushed

Salt & pepper to taste

Low cal cooking spray

Method:

Pre-heat the oven to 200C/fan 180C/gas 6.

Cook the barley until tender and drain. Spray the squash with low cal cooking oil and roast in the preheated oven for 20-25 minutes, or until tender.

Combine the olive oil, balsamic vinegar, Dijon mustard and garlic. Cook the broccoli into boiling salted water for 2-3 mins. Drain and combine with the barley, tomatoes, squash, olive oil dressing, olives, capers & watercress. Serve with chopped basil sprinkled over the top.

Soya Bean Salad

Serves: 1 Calories: 291

Ingredients:

40g/1½oz puy lentils

1 tsp each sesame oil & honey

1 tbsp lemon juice

½ garlic clove, crushed

½ tsp ground ginger & ¼ tsp crushed chilli flakes

2 tbsp soy sauce

250ml/1 cup vegetable stock/broth

2 stalks of tender stem broccoli, roughly chopped

40g/1½oz each fresh soya beans & sugar snap peas

1 tbsp fresh chopped oregano

Salt & pepper to taste

Method:

Make sure the stock is boiling hot and add the puy lentils. Cook for approx. 15 minutes or until tender, then drain. Meanwhile, add the broccoli, soya beans and sugar snap peas to a pan of boiling salted water and cook for 1-2 minutes until al dente. Drain and add to the cooling puy lentils. In a bowl, combine the sesame oil, honey, chilli flakes, lemon juice, garlic, ginger and soy sauce. Tip onto the lentil mix and combine gently to coat everything with the dressing. Season and serve with the chopped oregano over the top.

Fresh Herb Pitta

Serves: 1 Calories: 292

Ingredients:

150g/5oz frozen broad beans

½ cucumber

2 mini wholemeal pitta breads

1 tbsp lemon juice

1 tsp olive oil

Pinch caster sugar

1 tbsp fresh chopped mint

1 tbsp fresh chopped flat leaf parsley

1 tbsp fresh chopped chives

Method:

Combine together the lemon juice, olive oil, sugar and seasoning.

Chop the cucumber into small cubes. Cook the broad beans in a pan of salted boiling water for approx. 3 minutes or until tender; drain and leave to cool. Add the chopped cucumber to the beans in a shallow bowl and combine with the dressing. Cut the mini pitta breads into diagonal strips and arrange in the bowl with the beans. Serve sprinkled with the mint, parsley & chives.

Halloumi Water Melon Salad

Serves: 1 Calories: 277

Ingredients:

50g/2oz halloumi cheese, thinly sliced

250g/9oz watermelon flesh, cubed

50g/2oz fresh peas

75g/3oz baby courgettes/zucchini

1 tbsp lemon juice

1 tsp olive oil

1 tbsp chopped fresh mint

½ tsp crushed chilli flakes

Method:

Preheat the grill to medium/high.

Slice the baby courgettes lengthways and place on the grill, flesh side up, beside the sliced halloumi cheese. Season both well, sprinkle with chilli flakes and spray with a little low cal cooking spray.

Grill for 2-3 minutes each side or until golden. In a bowl mix together the mint, olive oil, cubed watermelon, fresh peas (eat these raw) and lemon juice. Arrange on a plate with the cheese and courgettes/zucchini.

Spicy Coconut Potatoes

Serves: 1 Calories: 246

Ingredients:

½ onion, chopped

75g/3oz potatoes, peeled and cubed

½ aubergine/egg plant, cubed

120g/4oz mushrooms, sliced

2 tsp curry powder

½ tsp paprika

60ml/¼ cup vegetable stock

60ml/ ¼ cup low fat coconut milk

1 tbsp fresh chopped coriander/cilantro

Low cal cooking spray

Method:

Gently sauté the onion in a little low cal cooking spray for a few minutes. Add the curry powder and paprika to a little water to make a paste and add this to the onions cooking in the pan. Add the potatoes and stock; cover and leave to simmer for a few minutes. Add the mushrooms and aubergine and cook for a further few minutes until everything is tender. Add the coconut milk and warm through. Serve with the chopped coriander sprinkled on top.

Moroccan Spinach Chickpeas

Serves: 1 Calories: 270

Ingredients:

1 onion, chopped

125g/4oz courgettes/zucchini, sliced

¼ tsp each ground cinnamon, turmeric, coriander/cilantro and cumin

1 fresh tomato, chopped

100g/3 ½ oz tinned chickpeas

Large handful of spinach, chopped

1 tbsp raisins

120ml/½ cup vegetable stock/broth

75g/3oz frozen peas

1 tbsp fresh chopped mint

Salt & pepper to taste

Low cal cooking spray

Method:

Gently sauté the onion and courgettes in a little low cal spray for a few minutes. Stir in the dried spices and chopped tomato; mix well. Season and add the chickpeas, raisins, peas and stock. Cover and leave to simmer for 5-10 minutes or until everything is tender and warmed through. Stir in the spinach and cook for a further minute. Sprinkle with fresh mint and serve.

Pea & Mint Risotto

Serves: 1 Calories: 277

Ingredients:

½ onion, chopped

75g/3oz frozen peas

370ml/1 ½ cups vegetable stock/broth

50g/3oz risotto rice

1 tsp grated Parmesan cheese

1 tbsp chopped fresh mint

Salt & pepper to taste

Low cal cooking spray

Method:

Gently sauté the onion in a little low cal cooking spray for a few minutes. Add the risotto rice and stir well. Add about a quarter of the stock to the rice, stirring and allowing the rice to absorb before adding more. Add the peas and chopped mint; keep on going for about 15 minutes until the risotto is tender and all the stock has been absorbed. Season, sprinkle with parmesan and serve.

Pasta Salad

Serves: 1 Calories: 289

Ingredients:

50g/3oz fusilli pasta

50g/2oz frozen peas

5 chopped black olives, finely chopped (optional)

2 chopped sundried tomatoes, finely chopped (optional)

1 tbsp balsamic vinegar

1 tbsp fresh chopped flat leaf parsley

1 tbsp lemon juice

2 tsp low fat mayo

Method:

Cook the fusilli in boiling salted water until tender, add the peas to the pan 5 minutes before the end of cooking time. Drain and leave to cool. Mix together the black olives, tomatoes, vinegar, mayonnaise and lemon juice to make a creamy dressing. Season and combine with the cooling pasta and peas. Serve with chopped parsley sprinkled over the top.

Egg & Mushroom Hash

Serves: 1 Calories: 286

Ingredients:

125g/4oz potatoes, diced

½ onion, chopped

½ tsp crushed chilli flakes

1 tsp olive oil

1 tsp dried basil or rosemary

50g/2oz mushrooms, chopped

1 medium free range egg

Method:

Pre-heat the oven to 180C/350f/gas 4. Mix the chopped onion, potato and mushrooms in a bowl with the olive oil, seasoning, chilli flakes and dried herbs. Spread out into a small shallow ovenproof dish and cook for 15-20 minutes or until the potatoes are tender. Make a 'well' in the middle of the potatoes and crack the egg in. Return to the oven and cook for another few minutes until the egg is cooked as you like it. Eat straight out of the oven dish.

Wholemeal, Cottage Cheese & Peppers

Serves: 1 Calories: 240

Ingredients:

75g/3oz low fat cottage cheese

½ red pepper, sliced

1 tsp chopped fresh basil leaves

2 slices wholemeal bread

1 tsp balsamic vinegar

Low cal cooking spray

Method:

Gently sauté the peppers in a little low cal cooking spray. Season and add the balsamic vinegar. Increase the heat so that the vinegar reduces and the peppers become sticky. Toast the bread and plate up with the cottage cheese on top. Tip the peppers and balsamic juice on the top, sprinkle with basil and serve.

Spring Chicken Stew

Serves: 1 Calories: 286

Ingredients:

100g/3 ½oz chicken breast, cubed

½ onion, chopped

1 carrot, finely chopped

1 celery stalk, finely chopped

½ tsp dried thyme

50g/2oz tender spring greens, shredded

250ml/1 cup chicken stock/broth

50g/2oz tinned haricot beans

1 tbsp chopped basil

Low cal cooking spray

Salt & pepper to taste

Method:

Put a frying pan on a high heat. Add a little low cal cooking spray and brown the chicken for a few minutes. Reduce the heat and add the onion, carrot, celery, thyme and stock. Cover and leave to gently simmer for 20-30 minutes or until the chicken is cooked through and the vegetables tender. Add the haricot beans and shredded greens; cook for a further few minutes. Season and serve with the chopped basil.

Chicken & Mango Noodles

Serves: 1 Calories: 230

Ingredients:

3 spring onions/scallions, chopped

½ tsp ground ginger

½ ripe mango, sliced

75g/3oz chicken breasts

100g/3½oz fresh stir-fry vegetables

1 tbsp soy sauce

1 tsp sweet chilli sauce

50g/2oz shirataki 'miracle' noodles

½ red chilli & ½ clove garlic, finely sliced

Low cal cooking spray

Salt & pepper to taste

Method:

Slice the chicken breast into strips. Put a frying pan on a high heat, add a little low cal cooking spray and stir-fry the chicken for a few minutes until cooked through. Meanwhile cook the shirataki noodles in salted boiling water as per the manufacturer's instructions.

Add the ginger, garlic, chilli and sweet chilli sauce to the chicken and stir-fry for a minute longer. Add the vegetables, spring onions, soy sauce, mango and noodles. Stir-fry for 2-3 minutes, season and serve.

Chicken Lettuce Bowls

Serves: 1 Calories: 266

Ingredients:

Zest of 1 lemon

1 garlic clove, 1 red chilli & 2 shallots, chopped

125g/4oz chicken breast, finely chopped

1 tsp sesame oil

½ tsp each paprika & ground ginger

1 tbsp each lime juice & fish sauce

50g/2oz bean sprouts

1 tbsp each fresh chopped mint & basil

1 baby gem lettuce, leaves peeled and left whole

Salt & pepper to taste

Low cal cooking spray

Method:

Mix the chillies, garlic, fish sauce, and lemon zest together with the sesame oil. Use a frying pan and a little low cal spray to cook the chicken on a high heat for a few minutes. Add the sesame oil dressing, paprika, ginger, bean sprouts, shallots and seasoning. Cook for a few minutes more until the chicken is cooked through. Remove from the heat, add the lime juice and chopped herbs and stir well. Arrange the lettuce leaves on a plate and divide the meat mixture into the lettuce leaves. Use your hands to pick each lettuce 'bowl' up to eat.

Mustard Chicken

Serves: 1 Calories: 293

Ingredients:

125g/4oz chicken breast

25g/1oz low fat grated cheddar cheese

1 tsp wholegrain mustard

2 tbsp single cream

1 tbsp milk

50g/2oz cherry tomatoes, halved

50g/2oz purple sprouting broccoli

Salt & pepper to taste

Low cal cooking spray

Method:

Pre-heat the oven to 200C/gas 6/fan 180C.

Cut the chicken through the middle to create two thinner breasts. Season and spray with a little low cal cooking oil; lay side by side in a small ovenproof dish. Mix together the cream, milk, grated cheese and mustard and spread onto the top of the chicken breasts. Season the tomatoes and place in the dish along with the chicken. Cook in the oven for 20-25 minutes or until the chicken is cooked through. 5 minutes before the end of cooking plunge the broccoli into boiling salted water and cook for 2-3 minutes. Drain and arrange on a plate along with the cooked chicken and cherry tomatoes.

Porcini Chicken & 'Rice'

Serves: 1 Calories: 296

Ingredients:

100g/3½ oz chicken breast, cubed

1 slice lean trimmed bacon, chopped

½ onion, chopped

1 garlic cloves, crushed

1 tbsp balsamic vinegar

60ml/¼ cup chicken stock/broth

1 tbsp dried porcini mushrooms, rehydrated and finely chopped

¼ head cauliflower

Salt & Pepper to taste

1 tbsp chopped fresh flat leaf parsley

Low cal cooking spray

Method:

In a food processor whizz the cauliflower until it is the size of rice grains. Use a frying pan to cook the chopped bacon and chicken in a little low cal cooking spray. Add the onion, stock, vinegar, porcini mushrooms and garlic to the pan; stir and season well. Cook for 3 minutes and add the cauliflower 'rice'. Cook until the liquid is reduced, the chicken cooked and the cauliflower tender. Serve sprinkled with flat leaf parsley.

Chicken & Avocado

Serves: 1 Calories: 295

Ingredients:

125g/4oz chicken breast

Pinch of paprika

¼ ripe avocado, diced

1 tsp red wine vinegar

1 tbsp balsamic vinegar

1 tsp fresh chopped chives

1 tomato, chopped

½ red onion chopped

1 baby gem lettuce, shredded

Salt & pepper to taste

Method:

Pre-heat a grill to medium/high. Season the chicken breast and cook for 10-12 minutes or until the chicken is cooked through. Meanwhile, mix together the vinegars and pour over the diced avocado, lettuce, chopped tomato and onion; toss well. When the chicken is cooked, cut into slices and serve over the top of the salad. Sprinkle the paprika and chives on top.

Chicken Couscous

Ingredients:

50g/2oz couscous

50g/2oz fresh peas

½ tsp dried basil

120ml/ ½ cup chicken stock/broth

100g/3½oz precooked breast

1 tomato, chopped

1 tbsp lemon juice

Method:

Place the couscous, dried basil and frozen peas into a bowl and pour the stock in; leave covered.

Meanwhile shred the cooked chicken and mix with the tomatoes and lemon juice; season well. After 4-6 minutes, check the couscous is tender and the peas cooked through. Drain any excess liquid and fluff with a fork. Toss in a bowl with the chicken and tomatoes.

Chicken & Spinach One Pot

Serves: 1 Calories: 297

Ingredients:

1 slice lean, back bacon, chopped

100g/3½oz chicken breast, cubed

50g/2oz mushrooms

1 tsp plain flour

150g/5oz tinned chopped tomatoes with garlic

½ beef stock cube

1 tsp Worcestershire sauce

1 tbsp fresh chopped chives

75g/3oz spinach leaves

Salt & pepper to taste

Low cal cooking spray

Method:

Place the flour in a plastic bag with the chicken and shake until the chicken is evenly coated with flour. In a frying pan, brown the bacon and chicken in a little low cal cooking spray for a few minutes. Add the rest of the ingredients, except the chives & spinach, Season well, cover and leave to cook for 8-10 minutes or until the chicken is cooked through. Add the spinach and serve with the chives sprinkled on top.

Sticky Chicken Noodles

Serves: 1 Calories: 288

Ingredients:

50g/2oz straight-to-wok or precooked egg noodles

1 tsp each honey & lemon juice

1 tbsp soy sauce

120ml/ ½ cup chicken stock/broth

75g/3oz chicken breast, cubed

1 tsp cornflour

50g/2oz courgette/zucchini, sliced

½ carrot and ¼ red pepper cut into matchsticks

Pinch of sesame seeds

Low cal cooking spray

Method:

Place the corn flour in a plastic bag with the chicken and shake until the chicken is evenly coated.

Brown the flour-coated chicken in a frying pan with a little low cal cooking spray for a few minutes. Meanwhile mix together the honey, lemon, stock and soy in a cup.

Add the carrots and peppers to the chicken and fry for a minute longer. Add the liquid in the cup to the pan, along with the noodles and courgettes/zucchini and cook for 5 minutes or until the chicken is properly cooked and the noodles warmed through. Serve straight away.

Chicken 'Pilau'

Serves: 1 Calories: 289

Ingredients:

100g/3½oz chicken breast, cubed

½ onion, chopped

1 clove garlic & ½ green chilli, finely chopped

½ tsp each ground ginger, cumin & turmeric

½ tsp ground coriander/cilantro

1 tbsp each lemon juice & fresh chopped coriander

125g/4oz tinned chopped tomatoes

½ head cauliflower

½ tsp sugar

Salt & pepper to taste

Low cal cooking spray

Method:

In a food processor whizz the cauliflower until it is the size of rice grains. Gently sauté the onion, garlic and chopped green chilli in a little low cal cooking spray for a few minutes. Add the chicken, lemon juice and dried spices and stir well. Add the tomatoes and sugar; season well.

Cover and leave to simmer for approx. 10 minutes or until the chicken is cooked through. Add the cauliflower rice and cook for a further 4-5 minutes (add a little water if needed). Check the cauliflower is tender and serve in a bowl with the chopped coriander sprinkled on top.

Chilli Steak & Broccoli Stir-Fry

Serves: 1 Calories: 256

Ingredients:

75g/3oz lean sirloin steak
1 clove garlic, crushed
½ tsp ground ginger
1 red chilli, deseeded and finely chopped
2 spring onion/scallions, sliced
125g/4oz tender stem broccoli, roughly chopped
2 tbsp soy sauce
100g/3½oz ready prepared stir-fry veg and beansprouts
Salt & pepper to taste
Low cal cooking spray

Method:

Season the steak and slice into small strips. Stir-fry in a little low cal cooking spray on a high heat. Add the garlic, ginger and chilli and cook for a minute longer, being careful not to burn the spices. Add the rest of the ingredients and continue to stir-fry for 2-3 minutes until the steak is cooked to your liking and the vegetables still nice and crunchy.

Chinese Garlic Beef

Serves: 1 Calories: 288

Ingredients:

100g/4oz lean sirloin steak

½ tsp Chinese five-spice

2 garlic cloves, crushed

2 spring onions/scallions, sliced

1 tbsp soy sauce

1 pak choi, shredded

40g/2oz mange tout

1 tsp sesame oil

Salt & pepper to taste

Low cal cooking spray

Method:

Mix the Chinese five-spice with a drop of water to make a paste and add the garlic.

Season the steak and brush with the garlic and spice mix. Put a little low cal cooking spray in a frying pan on a high heat and cook the steak for 2 minutes each side (longer if you like your meat well-done). Remove from the pan, leave to rest and then slice very thinly. Meanwhile, add a drop of water to the frying pan and add the pak choi, spring onion and mange tout along with the sesame oil. Stir-fry for a minute or two add the sliced steak back to the pan. Stir, season and serve.

Beef & Pineapple Salad

Serves: 1 Calories: 288

Ingredients:

75g/3oz beef fillet steak

2 tsp soy sauce & 1 tsp caster sugar

1 slice pineapple (fresh or tinned), finely chopped

1 carrot, cut into matchsticks

1 tbsp freshly chopped mint

1 tbsp each fish sauce & rice wine vinegar

2 garlic cloves & 1 red chilli, finely chopped

100g/3½oz rocket

2 tbsp pineapple juice

Method:

Mix one clove of garlic, ½ tsp sugar and the soy sauce together; brush onto the steak.

Mix together the other garlic clove, ½ tsp sugar, fish sauce, chopped chilli and pineapple juice to make a dressing.

Meanwhile fry the steak on a high heat in a dry pan for 2 minutes each side (more if you prefer well-done). Remove from the pan and rest.

Toss the pineapple juice dressing, rocket and carrots together. Slice the steak very thinly and place on top of the rocket mix. Sprinkle with chopped mint and serve.

Prawn Linguine

Serves: 1 Calories: 298

Ingredients:

50g/2oz linguine pasta

25g/1oz sugar snap peas

Handful of rocket

75g/3oz raw king prawns, peeled

1 garlic clove, crushed

½ red chilli, deseeded and finely chopped

4 cherry tomatoes, halved

1 tbsp fresh, chopped basil

1 tsp lime juice

½ tsp brown sugar

Salt & pepper to taste

Low cal cooking spray

Method:

Cook the linguine in boiling salted water until tender. Add the sugar snap peas to the pan 2 minutes before the end of cooking time. Drain and put to one side.

Meanwhile, gently cook the prawns, tomatoes, chilli and garlic in a little low cal cooking spray; season and stir through the lime juice and sugar. Ensure the prawns are fully cooked and toss into the pasta and mange tout. Sprinkle with chopped basil and serve.

Pak Choi Prawn Noodle Broth

Serves: 1 Calories: 294

Ingredients:

250ml/1 cup chicken stock/broth

75g/3oz raw king prawns, chopped

1 pak choi, chopped

50g/2oz straight-to-wok or precooked noodles

2 spring onions/scallions

2 tsp oyster sauce or hoisin sauce

1 tsp fish sauce

½ tsp ground ginger

Method:

Add all the ingredients, except the spring onions, to a wok. Gently simmer for 5-10 minutes or until the prawns are cooked through and the pak choi is wilted. Cut the spring onions lengthways into matchsticks. Tip the noodles into a bowl. Season and garnish with spring onion.

Salmon & Creamy Capers

Serves: 1 Calories: 291

Ingredients:

150g/5oz skinless salmon fillet

1 tbsp low fat crème fraîche

1 tbsp lemon juice

Large handful of spinach leaves

1 tsp capers, chopped

1 tbsp flat-leaf parsley, chopped

Low cal cooking spray

Method:

Season the salmon fillet then gently cook in a frying pan with a little low cal spray for approx. 6-8 minutes or until the fillet is cooked through. Leave to rest and add the spinach and lemon juice into the frying pan. Season well and stir for 1 minute until the spinach wilts. Place the salmon and spinach on a warmed plate and add the crème fraiche, capers and parsley to the pan, heat through gently and pour on top of the salmon fillet.

Smoked Salmon & Scrambled Eggs

Serves: 1 Calories: 288

Ingredients:

2 eggs

50g/2oz watercress

75g/3oz smoked salmon

1 lemon wedge

2 crackerbread

1 tsp low fat olive spread

Salt & pepper to taste

Method:

Crack the eggs into a cup, lightly whisk and season well. Arrange the smoked salmon slices on a plate with the lemon wedge; season with lots of black pepper. Use ½ tsp olive spread to 'butter' the crackerbread. Heat the other ½ tsp olive spread in a small frying pan and tip in the eggs. Keep on stirring continuously on a med/high heat until the eggs are nearly cooked but still 'sloppy'. Add the watercress; quickly stir through and serve with the salmon and crackerbread.

Chilli Mussels

Serves: 1 Calories: 253

Ingredients:

250g/9oz cleaned mussels
1 tomato, finely chopped
1 garlic clove, crushed
½ onion, chopped
120ml/½ cup dry white wine
120ml/½ cup fish or chicken stock
4 green olives, sliced
1 tsp dried chilli flakes
1 tbsp ketchup
1 tbsp freshly chopped basil leaves
Low cal cooking spray

Method:

In a pan sauté the garlic, olives, tomatoes, onions and
chilli in a little cooking spray. Add the wine, stock and
ketchup and stir well. Add the mussels, cover tightly and
steam for 3-5 minutes or until the mussels have opened.
(Throw away any which don't open). Tip everything into a
bowl. Sprinkle with basil leaves and serve.

Other CookNation Titles

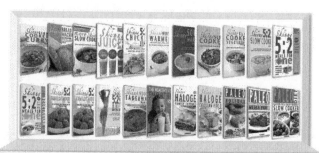

search cooknation on amazon to find all our titles

If you enjoyed *The Skinny 5:2 Diet Meals For One Recipe Book* we'd really appreciate your feedback. Reviews help others decide if this is the right book for them. Thank you.

You may also be interested in other titles in the CookNation series. Search 'CookNation' under Amazon.

7937949R00068

Printed in Great Britain
by Amazon.co.uk, Ltd.,
Marston Gate.